VET CONTROLLED SUBSTANCES LOG

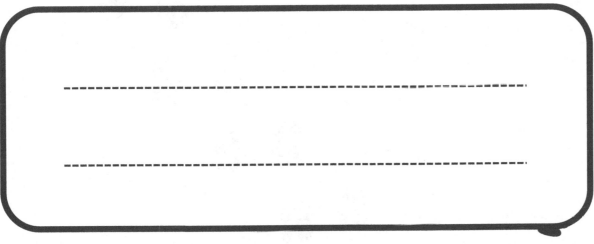

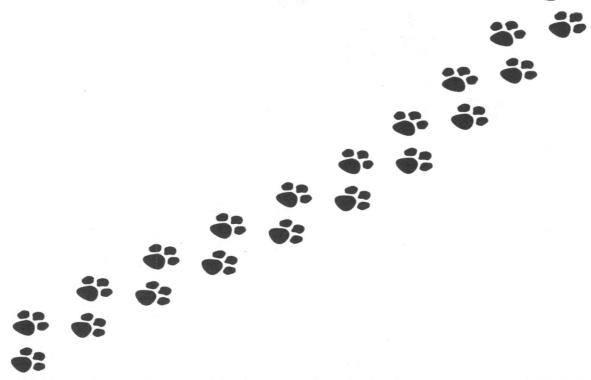

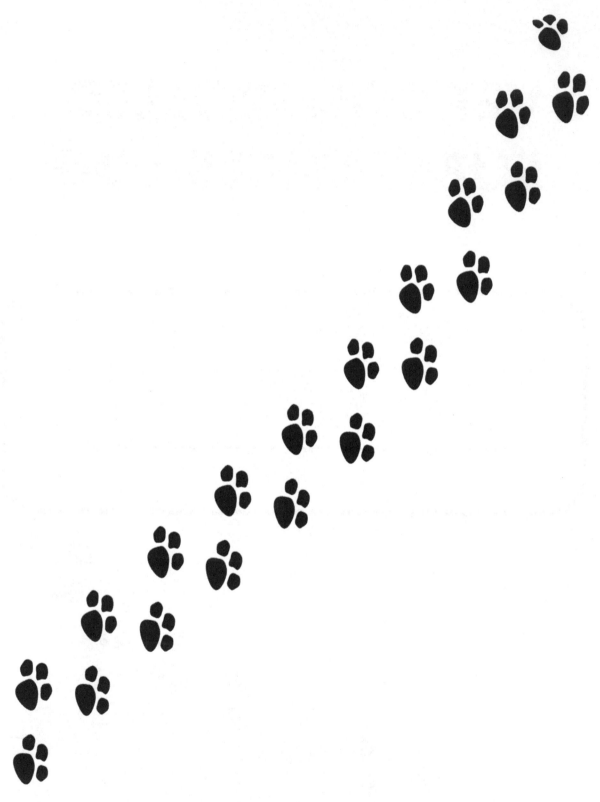

Bottle # : _____   Controlled Substance : _____

Serial # : _____   Class : _____

Expiration Date : _____   Concentration : _____

Container Size : _____   Form : _____

Date	Patient Name	Client ID	Initial Amount	Removed Amount	Remaining Amount	Authorized By	Dispensed By

Notes : _____

_____

_____

Bottle # : _____   **Controlled Substance :** _____

Serial # : _____   **Class :** _____

Expiration Date : _____   **Concentration :** _____

Container Size : _____   **Form :** _____

Date	Patient Name	Client ID	Initial Amount	Removed Amount	Remaining Amount	Authorized By	Dispensed By

Notes : _____

_____

_____

Bottle # : _____

Serial # : _____

Expiration Date : _____

Container Size : _____

Controlled Substance : _____

Class : _____

Concentration : _____

Form : _____

Date	Patient Name	Client ID	Initial Amount	Removed Amount	Remaining Amount	Authorized By	Dispensed By

Notes : _____

_____

_____

Bottle # : _____ Controlled Substance : _____

Serial # : _____ Class : _____

Expiration Date : _____ Concentration : _____

Container Size : _____ Form : _____

Date	Patient Name	Client ID	Initial Amount	Removed Amount	Remaining Amount	Authorized By	Dispensed By

Notes : _____

_____

_____

Bottle # : _____   Controlled Substance : _____

Serial # : _____   Class : _____

Expiration Date : _____   Concentration : _____

Container Size : _____   Form : _____

Date	Patient Name	Client ID	Initial Amount	Removed Amount	Remaining Amount	Authorized By	Dispensed By

Notes : _____

_____

_____

Bottle # : _____   Controlled Substance : _____

Serial # : _____   Class : _____

Expiration Date : _____   Concentration : _____

Container Size : _____   Form : _____

Date	Patient Name	Client ID	Initial Amount	Removed Amount	Remaining Amount	Authorized By	Dispensed By

Notes : _____

_____

_____

Bottle # : _____   Controlled Substance : _____

Serial # : _____   Class : _____

Expiration Date : _____   Concentration : _____

Container Size : _____   Form : _____

Date	Patient Name	Client ID	Initial Amount	Removed Amount	Remaining Amount	Authorized By	Dispensed By

Notes : _____

_____

_____

Bottle # : _____ Controlled Substance : _____

Serial # : _____ Class : _____

Expiration Date : _____ Concentration : _____

Container Size : _____ Form : _____

Date	Patient Name	Client ID	Initial Amount	Removed Amount	Remaining Amount	Authorized By	Dispensed By

Notes : _____

_____

_____

Bottle # : _____ Controlled Substance : _____

Serial # : _____ Class : _____

Expiration Date : _____ Concentration : _____

Container Size : _____ Form : _____

Date	Patient Name	Client ID	Initial Amount	Removed Amount	Remaining Amount	Authorized By	Dispensed By

Notes : _____

_____

_____

Bottle # : _____   **Controlled Substance :** _____

Serial # : _____   **Class :** _____

Expiration Date : _____   **Concentration :** _____

Container Size : _____   **Form :** _____

Date	Patient Name	Client ID	Initial Amount	Removed Amount	Remaining Amount	Authorized By	Dispensed By

Notes : _____

_____

_____

Bottle # : _____   Controlled Substance : _____

Serial # : _____   Class : _____

Expiration Date : _____   Concentration : _____

Container Size : _____   Form : _____

Date	Patient Name	Client ID	Initial Amount	Removed Amount	Remaining Amount	Authorized By	Dispensed By

Notes : _____

_____

_____

Bottle # : _____ Controlled Substance : _____

Serial # : _____ Class : _____

Expiration Date : _____ Concentration : _____

Container Size : _____ Form : _____

Date	Patient Name	Client ID	Initial Amount	Removed Amount	Remaining Amount	Authorized By	Dispensed By

Notes : _____

_____

_____

Bottle # : _____   Controlled Substance : _____

Serial # : _____   Class : _____

Expiration Date : _____   Concentration : _____

Container Size : _____   Form : _____

Date	Patient Name	Client ID	Initial Amount	Removed Amount	Remaining Amount	Authorized By	Dispensed By

Notes : _____

_____

_____

Bottle # : _____ **Controlled Substance :** _____

Serial # : _____ **Class :** _____

Expiration Date : _____ **Concentration :** _____

Container Size : _____ **Form :** _____

Date	Patient Name	Client ID	Initial Amount	Removed Amount	Remaining Amount	Authorized By	Dispensed By

Notes : _____

_____

_____

Bottle # : _____   Controlled Substance : _____

Serial # : _____   Class : _____

Expiration Date : _____   Concentration : _____

Container Size : _____   Form : _____

Date	Patient Name	Client ID	Initial Amount	Removed Amount	Remaining Amount	Authorized By	Dispensed By

Notes : _____

_____

_____

Bottle # : _____ **Controlled Substance :** _____

Serial # : _____ **Class :** _____

Expiration Date : _____ **Concentration :** _____

Container Size : _____ **Form :** _____

Date	Patient Name	Client ID	Initial Amount	Removed Amount	Remaining Amount	Authorized By	Dispensed By

Notes : _____

_____

_____

Bottle # : _____   Controlled Substance : _____

Serial # : _____   Class : _____

Expiration Date : _____   Concentration : _____

Container Size : _____   Form : _____

Date	Patient Name	Client ID	Initial Amount	Removed Amount	Remaining Amount	Authorized By	Dispensed By

Notes : _____

_____

_____

Bottle # : _____ **Controlled Substance :** _____

Serial # : _____ **Class :** _____

Expiration Date : _____ **Concentration :** _____

Container Size : _____ **Form :** _____

Date	Patient Name	Client ID	Initial Amount	Removed Amount	Remaining Amount	Authorized By	Dispensed By

Notes : _____

_____

_____

Bottle # : _____   Controlled Substance : _____

Serial # : _____   Class : _____

Expiration Date : _____   Concentration : _____

Container Size : _____   Form : _____

Date	Patient Name	Client ID	Initial Amount	Removed Amount	Remaining Amount	Authorized By	Dispensed By

Notes : _____

_____

_____

Bottle # : _____

Serial # : _____

Expiration Date : _____

Container Size : _____

Controlled Substance : _____

Class : _____

Concentration : _____

Form : _____

Date	Patient Name	Client ID	Initial Amount	Removed Amount	Remaining Amount	Authorized By	Dispensed By

Notes : _____

_____

_____

Bottle # : _____ Controlled Substance : _____

Serial # : _____ Class : _____

Expiration Date : _____ Concentration : _____

Container Size : _____ Form : _____

Date	Patient Name	Client ID	Initial Amount	Removed Amount	Remaining Amount	Authorized By	Dispensed By

Notes : _____

_____

_____

Bottle # : _____ Controlled Substance : _____

Serial # : _____ Class : _____

Expiration Date : _____ Concentration : _____

Container Size : _____ Form : _____

Date	Patient Name	Client ID	Initial Amount	Removed Amount	Remaining Amount	Authorized By	Dispensed By

Notes : _____

_____

_____

Bottle # : _____   Controlled Substance : _____

Serial # : _____   Class : _____

Expiration Date : _____   Concentration : _____

Container Size : _____   Form : _____

Date	Patient Name	Client ID	Initial Amount	Removed Amount	Remaining Amount	Authorized By	Dispensed By

Notes : _____

_____

_____

Bottle # : _____ Controlled Substance : _____

Serial # : _____ Class : _____

Expiration Date : _____ Concentration : _____

Container Size : _____ Form : _____

Date	Patient Name	Client ID	Initial Amount	Removed Amount	Remaining Amount	Authorized By	Dispensed By

Notes : _____

_____

_____

Bottle # : _____   Controlled Substance : _____

Serial # : _____   Class : _____

Expiration Date : _____   Concentration : _____

Container Size : _____   Form : _____

Date	Patient Name	Client ID	Initial Amount	Removed Amount	Remaining Amount	Authorized By	Dispensed By

Notes : _____

_____

_____

Bottle # : _____ **Controlled Substance :** _____

Serial # : _____ **Class :** _____

Expiration Date : _____ **Concentration :** _____

Container Size : _____ **Form :** _____

Date	Patient Name	Client ID	Initial Amount	Removed Amount	Remaining Amount	Authorized By	Dispensed By

Notes : _____

_____

_____

Bottle # : _____ Controlled Substance : _____

Serial # : _____ Class : _____

Expiration Date : _____ Concentration : _____

Container Size : _____ Form : _____

Date	Patient Name	Client ID	Initial Amount	Removed Amount	Remaining Amount	Authorized By	Dispensed By

Notes : _____

_____

_____

Bottle # : ....   Controlled Substance : ....

Serial # : ....   Class : ....

Expiration Date : ....   Concentration : ....

Container Size : ....   Form : ....

Date	Patient Name	Client ID	Initial Amount	Removed Amount	Remaining Amount	Authorized By	Dispensed By

Notes : ....

....

....

Bottle # : _____ Controlled Substance : _____

Serial # : _____ Class : _____

Expiration Date : _____ Concentration : _____

Container Size : _____ Form : _____

Date	Patient Name	Client ID	Initial Amount	Removed Amount	Remaining Amount	Authorized By	Dispensed By

Notes : _____

_____

_____

Bottle # : _____ Controlled Substance : _____

Serial # : _____ Class : _____

Expiration Date : _____ Concentration : _____

Container Size : _____ Form : _____

Date	Patient Name	Client ID	Initial Amount	Removed Amount	Remaining Amount	Authorized By	Dispensed By

Notes : _____

_____

_____

_____

Bottle # : _____   Controlled Substance : _____

Serial # : _____   Class : _____

Expiration Date : _____   Concentration : _____

Container Size : _____   Form : _____

Date	Patient Name	Client ID	Initial Amount	Removed Amount	Remaining Amount	Authorized By	Dispensed By

Notes : _____

_____

_____

Bottle # : _____ **Controlled Substance :** _____

Serial # : _____ **Class :** _____

Expiration Date : _____ **Concentration :** _____

Container Size : _____ **Form :** _____

Date	Patient Name	Client ID	Initial Amount	Removed Amount	Remaining Amount	Authorized By	Dispensed By

Notes : _____

_____

_____

Bottle # : _____ Controlled Substance : _____

Serial # : _____ Class : _____

Expiration Date : _____ Concentration : _____

Container Size : _____ Form : _____

Date	Patient Name	Client ID	Initial Amount	Removed Amount	Remaining Amount	Authorized By	Dispensed By

Notes : _____

_____

_____

Bottle # : _____   **Controlled Substance :** _____

Serial # : _____   **Class :** _____

Expiration Date : _____   **Concentration :** _____

Container Size : _____   **Form :** _____

Date	Patient Name	Client ID	Initial Amount	Removed Amount	Remaining Amount	Authorized By	Dispensed By

Notes : _____

_____

_____

Bottle # : _____   Controlled Substance : _____

Serial # : _____   Class : _____

Expiration Date : _____   Concentration : _____

Container Size : _____   Form : _____

Date	Patient Name	Client ID	Initial Amount	Removed Amount	Remaining Amount	Authorized By	Dispensed By

Notes : _____

_____

_____

Bottle # : _____   Controlled Substance : _____

Serial # : _____   Class : _____

Expiration Date : _____   Concentration : _____

Container Size : _____   Form : _____

Date	Patient Name	Client ID	Initial Amount	Removed Amount	Remaining Amount	Authorized By	Dispensed By

Notes : _____

_____

_____

Bottle # : _____   Controlled Substance : _____

Serial # : _____   Class : _____

Expiration Date : _____   Concentration : _____

Container Size : _____   Form : _____

Date	Patient Name	Client ID	Initial Amount	Removed Amount	Remaining Amount	Authorized By	Dispensed By

Notes : _____

_____

_____

Bottle # : _____   Controlled Substance : _____

Serial # : _____   Class : _____

Expiration Date : _____   Concentration : _____

Container Size : _____   Form : _____

Date	Patient Name	Client ID	Initial Amount	Removed Amount	Remaining Amount	Authorized By	Dispensed By

Notes : _____

_____

_____

Bottle # : _____   Controlled Substance : _____

Serial # : _____   Class : _____

Expiration Date : _____   Concentration : _____

Container Size : _____   Form : _____

Date	Patient Name	Client ID	Initial Amount	Removed Amount	Remaining Amount	Authorized By	Dispensed By

Notes : _____

_____

_____

Bottle # : ....

Serial # : ....

Expiration Date : ....

Container Size : ....

Controlled Substance : ....

Class : ....

Concentration : ....

Form : ....

Date	Patient Name	Client ID	Initial Amount	Removed Amount	Remaining Amount	Authorized By	Dispensed By

Notes : ....

....

....

Bottle # : _____   Controlled Substance : _____

Serial # : _____   Class : _____

Expiration Date : _____   Concentration : _____

Container Size : _____   Form : _____

Date	Patient Name	Client ID	Initial Amount	Removed Amount	Remaining Amount	Authorized By	Dispensed By

Notes : _____

_____

_____

Bottle # : _____

Serial # : _____

Expiration Date : _____

Container Size : _____

Controlled Substance : _____

Class : _____

Concentration : _____

Form : _____

Date	Patient Name	Client ID	Initial Amount	Removed Amount	Remaining Amount	Authorized By	Dispensed By

Notes : _____

_____

_____

Bottle # : _____   Controlled Substance : _____

Serial # : _____   Class : _____

Expiration Date : _____   Concentration : _____

Container Size : _____   Form : _____

Date	Patient Name	Client ID	Initial Amount	Removed Amount	Remaining Amount	Authorized By	Dispensed By

Notes : _____

_____

_____

Bottle # : ....

Serial # : ....

Expiration Date : ....

Container Size : ....

Controlled Substance : ....

Class : ....

Concentration : ....

Form : ....

Date	Patient Name	Client ID	Initial Amount	Removed Amount	Remaining Amount	Authorized By	Dispensed By

Notes : ....

....

....

Bottle # : _____   Controlled Substance : _____

Serial # : _____   Class : _____

Expiration Date : _____   Concentration : _____

Container Size : _____   Form : _____

Date	Patient Name	Client ID	Initial Amount	Removed Amount	Remaining Amount	Authorized By	Dispensed By

Notes : _____

_____

_____

Bottle # : _____ Controlled Substance : _____

Serial # : _____ Class : _____

Expiration Date : _____ Concentration : _____

Container Size : _____ Form : _____

Date	Patient Name	Client ID	Initial Amount	Removed Amount	Remaining Amount	Authorized By	Dispensed By

Notes : _____

_____

_____

Bottle # : _____ Controlled Substance : _____

Serial # : _____ Class : _____

Expiration Date : _____ Concentration : _____

Container Size : _____ Form : _____

Date	Patient Name	Client ID	Initial Amount	Removed Amount	Remaining Amount	Authorized By	Dispensed By

Notes : _____

_____

_____

Bottle # : _____   **Controlled Substance :** _____

Serial # : _____   **Class :** _____

Expiration Date : _____   **Concentration :** _____

Container Size : _____   **Form :** _____

Date	Patient Name	Client ID	Initial Amount	Removed Amount	Remaining Amount	Authorized By	Dispensed By

Notes : _____

_____

_____

Bottle # : _____   Controlled Substance : _____

Serial # : _____   Class : _____

Expiration Date : _____   Concentration : _____

Container Size : _____   Form : _____

Date	Patient Name	Client ID	Initial Amount	Removed Amount	Remaining Amount	Authorized By	Dispensed By

Notes : _____

_____

_____

Bottle # : _____ **Controlled Substance :** _____

Serial # : _____ **Class :** _____

Expiration Date : _____ **Concentration :** _____

Container Size : _____ **Form :** _____

Date	Patient Name	Client ID	Initial Amount	Removed Amount	Remaining Amount	Authorized By	Dispensed By

Notes : _____

_____

_____

_____

Bottle # : _____   **Controlled Substance :** _____

Serial # : _____   **Class :** _____

Expiration Date : _____   **Concentration :** _____

Container Size : _____   **Form :** _____

Date	Patient Name	Client ID	Initial Amount	Removed Amount	Remaining Amount	Authorized By	Dispensed By

Notes : _____

_____

_____

Bottle # : _____ Controlled Substance : _____

Serial # : _____ Class : _____

Expiration Date : _____ Concentration : _____

Container Size : _____ Form : _____

Date	Patient Name	Client ID	Initial Amount	Removed Amount	Remaining Amount	Authorized By	Dispensed By

Notes : _____

_____

_____

Bottle # : _____   Controlled Substance : _____

Serial # : _____   Class : _____

Expiration Date : _____   Concentration : _____

Container Size : _____   Form : _____

Date	Patient Name	Client ID	Initial Amount	Removed Amount	Remaining Amount	Authorized By	Dispensed By

Notes : _____

_____

_____

Bottle # : _____ **Controlled Substance :** _____

Serial # : _____ **Class :** _____

Expiration Date : _____ **Concentration :** _____

Container Size : _____ **Form :** _____

Date	Patient Name	Client ID	Initial Amount	Removed Amount	Remaining Amount	Authorized By	Dispensed By

Notes : _____

_____

_____

Bottle # : _____   Controlled Substance : _____

Serial # : _____   Class : _____

Expiration Date : _____   Concentration : _____

Container Size : _____   Form : _____

Date	Patient Name	Client ID	Initial Amount	Removed Amount	Remaining Amount	Authorized By	Dispensed By

Notes : _____

_____

_____

Bottle # : _____ **Controlled Substance :** _____

Serial # : _____ **Class :** _____

Expiration Date : _____ **Concentration :** _____

Container Size : _____ **Form :** _____

Date	Patient Name	Client ID	Initial Amount	Removed Amount	Remaining Amount	Authorized By	Dispensed By

Notes : _____

_____

_____

Bottle # : _____ Controlled Substance : _____

Serial # : _____ Class : _____

Expiration Date : _____ Concentration : _____

Container Size : _____ Form : _____

Date	Patient Name	Client ID	Initial Amount	Removed Amount	Remaining Amount	Authorized By	Dispensed By

Notes : _____

_____

_____

Bottle # : _____ Controlled Substance : _____

Serial # : _____ Class : _____

Expiration Date : _____ Concentration : _____

Container Size : _____ Form : _____

Date	Patient Name	Client ID	Initial Amount	Removed Amount	Remaining Amount	Authorized By	Dispensed By

Notes : _____

_____

_____

Bottle # : _____   Controlled Substance : _____

Serial # : _____   Class : _____

Expiration Date : _____   Concentration : _____

Container Size : _____   Form : _____

Date	Patient Name	Client ID	Initial Amount	Removed Amount	Remaining Amount	Authorized By	Dispensed By

Notes : _____

_____

_____

Bottle # : _____ Controlled Substance : _____

Serial # : _____ Class : _____

Expiration Date : _____ Concentration : _____

Container Size : _____ Form : _____

Date	Patient Name	Client ID	Initial Amount	Removed Amount	Remaining Amount	Authorized By	Dispensed By

Notes : _____

_____

_____

Bottle # : _____ Controlled Substance : _____

Serial # : _____ Class : _____

Expiration Date : _____ Concentration : _____

Container Size : _____ Form : _____

Date	Patient Name	Client ID	Initial Amount	Removed Amount	Remaining Amount	Authorized By	Dispensed By

Notes : _____

_____

_____

Bottle # : _____   Controlled Substance : _____

Serial # : _____   Class : _____

Expiration Date : _____   Concentration : _____

Container Size : _____   Form : _____

Date	Patient Name	Client ID	Initial Amount	Removed Amount	Remaining Amount	Authorized By	Dispensed By

Notes : _____

_____

_____

_____

Bottle # : _____   Controlled Substance : _____

Serial # : _____   Class : _____

Expiration Date : _____   Concentration : _____

Container Size : _____   Form : _____

Date	Patient Name	Client ID	Initial Amount	Removed Amount	Remaining Amount	Authorized By	Dispensed By

Notes : _____
_____
_____

Bottle # : _____   Controlled Substance : _____

Serial # : _____   Class : _____

Expiration Date : _____   Concentration : _____

Container Size : _____   Form : _____

Date	Patient Name	Client ID	Initial Amount	Removed Amount	Remaining Amount	Authorized By	Dispensed By

Notes : _____

_____

_____

Bottle # : _____   Controlled Substance : _____

Serial # : _____   Class : _____

Expiration Date : _____   Concentration : _____

Container Size : _____   Form : _____

Date	Patient Name	Client ID	Initial Amount	Removed Amount	Remaining Amount	Authorized By	Dispensed By

Notes : _____

_____

_____

Bottle # : _____ Controlled Substance : _____

Serial # : _____ Class : _____

Expiration Date : _____ Concentration : _____

Container Size : _____ Form : _____

Date	Patient Name	Client ID	Initial Amount	Removed Amount	Remaining Amount	Authorized By	Dispensed By

Notes : _____

_____

_____

Bottle # : _____   Controlled Substance : _____

Serial # : _____   Class : _____

Expiration Date : _____   Concentration : _____

Container Size : _____   Form : _____

Date	Patient Name	Client ID	Initial Amount	Removed Amount	Remaining Amount	Authorized By	Dispensed By

Notes : _____

_____

_____

Bottle # : _____   Controlled Substance : _____

Serial # : _____   Class : _____

Expiration Date : _____   Concentration : _____

Container Size : _____   Form : _____

Date	Patient Name	Client ID	Initial Amount	Removed Amount	Remaining Amount	Authorized By	Dispensed By

Notes : _____

_____

_____

Bottle # : _____   Controlled Substance : _____

Serial # : _____   Class : _____

Expiration Date : _____   Concentration : _____

Container Size : _____   Form : _____

Date	Patient Name	Client ID	Initial Amount	Removed Amount	Remaining Amount	Authorized By	Dispensed By

Notes : _____

_____

_____

Bottle # : _____ Controlled Substance : _____

Serial # : _____ Class : _____

Expiration Date : _____ Concentration : _____

Container Size : _____ Form : _____

Date	Patient Name	Client ID	Initial Amount	Removed Amount	Remaining Amount	Authorized By	Dispensed By

Notes : _____

_____

_____

Bottle # : _____   Controlled Substance : _____

Serial # : _____   Class : _____

Expiration Date : _____   Concentration : _____

Container Size : _____   Form : _____

Date	Patient Name	Client ID	Initial Amount	Removed Amount	Remaining Amount	Authorized By	Dispensed By

Notes : _____

_____

_____

Bottle # : _____   Controlled Substance : _____

Serial # : _____   Class : _____

Expiration Date : _____   Concentration : _____

Container Size : _____   Form : _____

Date	Patient Name	Client ID	Initial Amount	Removed Amount	Remaining Amount	Authorized By	Dispensed By

Notes : _____

_____

_____

Bottle # : _____ Controlled Substance : _____

Serial # : _____ Class : _____

Expiration Date : _____ Concentration : _____

Container Size : _____ Form : _____

Date	Patient Name	Client ID	Initial Amount	Removed Amount	Remaining Amount	Authorized By	Dispensed By

Notes : _____

_____

_____

Bottle # : _____ Controlled Substance : _____

Serial # : _____ Class : _____

Expiration Date : _____ Concentration : _____

Container Size : _____ Form : _____

Date	Patient Name	Client ID	Initial Amount	Removed Amount	Remaining Amount	Authorized By	Dispensed By

Notes : _____

_____

_____

Bottle # : _____ Controlled Substance : _____

Serial # : _____ Class : _____

Expiration Date : _____ Concentration : _____

Container Size : _____ Form : _____

Date	Patient Name	Client ID	Initial Amount	Removed Amount	Remaining Amount	Authorized By	Dispensed By

Notes : _____

_____

_____

Bottle # : ....

Serial # : ....

Expiration Date : ....

Container Size : ....

Controlled Substance : ....

Class : ....

Concentration : ....

Form : ....

Date	Patient Name	Client ID	Initial Amount	Removed Amount	Remaining Amount	Authorized By	Dispensed By

Notes : ....

....

....

Bottle # : _____ Controlled Substance : _____

Serial # : _____ Class : _____

Expiration Date : _____ Concentration : _____

Container Size : _____ Form : _____

Date	Patient Name	Client ID	Initial Amount	Removed Amount	Remaining Amount	Authorized By	Dispensed By

Notes : _____

_____

_____

Bottle # : _____   Controlled Substance : _____

Serial # : _____   Class : _____

Expiration Date : _____   Concentration : _____

Container Size : _____   Form : _____

Date	Patient Name	Client ID	Initial Amount	Removed Amount	Remaining Amount	Authorized By	Dispensed By

Notes : _____

_____

_____

Bottle # : _____ Controlled Substance : _____

Serial # : _____ Class : _____

Expiration Date : _____ Concentration : _____

Container Size : _____ Form : _____

Date	Patient Name	Client ID	Initial Amount	Removed Amount	Remaining Amount	Authorized By	Dispensed By

Notes : _____

_____

_____

Bottle # : _____ Controlled Substance : _____

Serial # : _____ Class : _____

Expiration Date : _____ Concentration : _____

Container Size : _____ Form : _____

Date	Patient Name	Client ID	Initial Amount	Removed Amount	Remaining Amount	Authorized By	Dispensed By

Notes : _____

_____

_____

_____

Bottle # : _____   Controlled Substance : _____

Serial # : _____   Class : _____

Expiration Date : _____   Concentration : _____

Container Size : _____   Form : _____

Date	Patient Name	Client ID	Initial Amount	Removed Amount	Remaining Amount	Authorized By	Dispensed By

Notes : _____

_____

_____

Bottle # : _____ Controlled Substance : _____

Serial # : _____ Class : _____

Expiration Date : _____ Concentration : _____

Container Size : _____ Form : _____

Date	Patient Name	Client ID	Initial Amount	Removed Amount	Remaining Amount	Authorized By	Dispensed By

Notes : _____
_____
_____
_____

Bottle # : _____   Controlled Substance : _____

Serial # : _____   Class : _____

Expiration Date : _____   Concentration : _____

Container Size : _____   Form : _____

Date	Patient Name	Client ID	Initial Amount	Removed Amount	Remaining Amount	Authorized By	Dispensed By

Notes : _____

_____

_____

Bottle # : _____   **Controlled Substance :** _____

Serial # : _____   **Class :** _____

Expiration Date : _____   **Concentration :** _____

Container Size : _____   **Form :** _____

Date	Patient Name	Client ID	Initial Amount	Removed Amount	Remaining Amount	Authorized By	Dispensed By

Notes : _____

_____

_____

Bottle # : _____   Controlled Substance : _____

Serial # : _____   Class : _____

Expiration Date : _____   Concentration : _____

Container Size : _____   Form : _____

Date	Patient Name	Client ID	Initial Amount	Removed Amount	Remaining Amount	Authorized By	Dispensed By

Notes : _____

_____

_____

Bottle # : _____ Controlled Substance : _____

Serial # : _____ Class : _____

Expiration Date : _____ Concentration : _____

Container Size : _____ Form : _____

Date	Patient Name	Client ID	Initial Amount	Removed Amount	Remaining Amount	Authorized By	Dispensed By

Notes : _____

_____

_____

Bottle # : _____   Controlled Substance : _____

Serial # : _____   Class : _____

Expiration Date : _____   Concentration : _____

Container Size : _____   Form : _____

Date	Patient Name	Client ID	Initial Amount	Removed Amount	Remaining Amount	Authorized By	Dispensed By

Notes : _____

_____

_____

Bottle # : _____   Controlled Substance : _____

Serial # : _____   Class : _____

Expiration Date : _____   Concentration : _____

Container Size : _____   Form : _____

Date	Patient Name	Client ID	Initial Amount	Removed Amount	Remaining Amount	Authorized By	Dispensed By

Notes : _____

_____

_____

Bottle # : _____   Controlled Substance : _____

Serial # : _____   Class : _____

Expiration Date : _____   Concentration : _____

Container Size : _____   Form : _____

Date	Patient Name	Client ID	Initial Amount	Removed Amount	Remaining Amount	Authorized By	Dispensed By

Notes : _____

_____

_____

Bottle # : _____ Controlled Substance : _____

Serial # : _____ Class : _____

Expiration Date : _____ Concentration : _____

Container Size : _____ Form : _____

Date	Patient Name	Client ID	Initial Amount	Removed Amount	Remaining Amount	Authorized By	Dispensed By

Notes : _____

_____

_____

Bottle # : _____   Controlled Substance : _____

Serial # : _____   Class : _____

Expiration Date : _____   Concentration : _____

Container Size : _____   Form : _____

Date	Patient Name	Client ID	Initial Amount	Removed Amount	Remaining Amount	Authorized By	Dispensed By

Notes : _____

_____

_____

Bottle # : _____   Controlled Substance : _____

Serial # : _____   Class : _____

Expiration Date : _____   Concentration : _____

Container Size : _____   Form : _____

Date	Patient Name	Client ID	Initial Amount	Removed Amount	Remaining Amount	Authorized By	Dispensed By

Notes : _____

_____

_____

Bottle # : _____ Controlled Substance : _____

Serial # : _____ Class : _____

Expiration Date : _____ Concentration : _____

Container Size : _____ Form : _____

Date	Patient Name	Client ID	Initial Amount	Removed Amount	Remaining Amount	Authorized By	Dispensed By

Notes : _____

_____

_____

Bottle # : _____ Controlled Substance : _____

Serial # : _____ Class : _____

Expiration Date : _____ Concentration : _____

Container Size : _____ Form : _____

Date	Patient Name	Client ID	Initial Amount	Removed Amount	Remaining Amount	Authorized By	Dispensed By

Notes : _____

_____

_____

Bottle # : _____ Controlled Substance : _____

Serial # : _____ Class : _____

Expiration Date : _____ Concentration : _____

Container Size : _____ Form : _____

Date	Patient Name	Client ID	Initial Amount	Removed Amount	Remaining Amount	Authorized By	Dispensed By

Notes : _____

_____

_____

Bottle # : _____   Controlled Substance : _____

Serial # : _____   Class : _____

Expiration Date : _____   Concentration : _____

Container Size : _____   Form : _____

Date	Patient Name	Client ID	Initial Amount	Removed Amount	Remaining Amount	Authorized By	Dispensed By

Notes : _____

_____

_____

Bottle # : _____ Controlled Substance : _____

Serial # : _____ Class : _____

Expiration Date : _____ Concentration : _____

Container Size : _____ Form : _____

Date	Patient Name	Client ID	Initial Amount	Removed Amount	Remaining Amount	Authorized By	Dispensed By

Notes : _____

_____

_____

Bottle # : _____ **Controlled Substance :** _____

Serial # : _____ **Class :** _____

Expiration Date : _____ **Concentration :** _____

Container Size : _____ **Form :** _____

Date	Patient Name	Client ID	Initial Amount	Removed Amount	Remaining Amount	Authorized By	Dispensed By

Notes : _____

_____

_____

Bottle # : _____   Controlled Substance : _____

Serial # : _____   Class : _____

Expiration Date : _____   Concentration : _____

Container Size : _____   Form : _____

Date	Patient Name	Client ID	Initial Amount	Removed Amount	Remaining Amount	Authorized By	Dispensed By

Notes : _____

_____

_____

Bottle # : .... Controlled Substance : ....

Serial # : .... Class : ....

Expiration Date : .... Concentration : ....

Container Size : .... Form : ....

Date	Patient Name	Client ID	Initial Amount	Removed Amount	Remaining Amount	Authorized By	Dispensed By

Notes : ....

....

....

Bottle # : _____   Controlled Substance : _____

Serial # : _____   Class : _____

Expiration Date : _____   Concentration : _____

Container Size : _____   Form : _____

Date	Patient Name	Client ID	Initial Amount	Removed Amount	Remaining Amount	Authorized By	Dispensed By

Notes : _____

_____

_____

Bottle # : _____   Controlled Substance : _____

Serial # : _____   Class : _____

Expiration Date : _____   Concentration : _____

Container Size : _____   Form : _____

Date	Patient Name	Client ID	Initial Amount	Removed Amount	Remaining Amount	Authorized By	Dispensed By

Notes : _____

_____

_____

_____

Bottle # : _____   Controlled Substance : _____

Serial # : _____   Class : _____

Expiration Date : _____   Concentration : _____

Container Size : _____   Form : _____

Date	Patient Name	Client ID	Initial Amount	Removed Amount	Remaining Amount	Authorized By	Dispensed By

Notes : _____

_____

_____

Bottle # : _____   **Controlled Substance :** _____

Serial # : _____   **Class :** _____

Expiration Date : _____   **Concentration :** _____

Container Size : _____   **Form :** _____

Date	Patient Name	Client ID	Initial Amount	Removed Amount	Remaining Amount	Authorized By	Dispensed By

Notes : _____

_____

_____

Bottle # : _____   Controlled Substance : _____

Serial # : _____   Class : _____

Expiration Date : _____   Concentration : _____

Container Size : _____   Form : _____

Date	Patient Name	Client ID	Initial Amount	Removed Amount	Remaining Amount	Authorized By	Dispensed By

Notes : _____

_____

_____

Bottle # : _____   Controlled Substance : _____

Serial # : _____   Class : _____

Expiration Date : _____   Concentration : _____

Container Size : _____   Form : _____

Date	Patient Name	Client ID	Initial Amount	Removed Amount	Remaining Amount	Authorized By	Dispensed By

Notes : _____

_____

_____

Bottle # : _____ Controlled Substance : _____

Serial # : _____ Class : _____

Expiration Date : _____ Concentration : _____

Container Size : _____ Form : _____

Date	Patient Name	Client ID	Initial Amount	Removed Amount	Remaining Amount	Authorized By	Dispensed By

Notes : _____

_____

_____

Bottle # : .... Controlled Substance : ....

Serial # : .... Class : ....

Expiration Date : .... Concentration : ....

Container Size : .... Form : ....

Date	Patient Name	Client ID	Initial Amount	Removed Amount	Remaining Amount	Authorized By	Dispensed By

Notes : ....

....

....

Bottle # : _____ **Controlled Substance :** _____

Serial # : _____ **Class :** _____

Expiration Date : _____ **Concentration :** _____

Container Size : _____ **Form :** _____

Date	Patient Name	Client ID	Initial Amount	Removed Amount	Remaining Amount	Authorized By	Dispensed By

Notes : _____

_____

_____

Bottle # : _____ **Controlled Substance :** _____

Serial # : _____ **Class :** _____

Expiration Date : _____ **Concentration :** _____

Container Size : _____ **Form :** _____

Date	Patient Name	Client ID	Initial Amount	Removed Amount	Remaining Amount	Authorized By	Dispensed By

Notes : _____

_____

_____

Bottle # : _____   Controlled Substance : _____

Serial # : _____   Class : _____

Expiration Date : _____   Concentration : _____

Container Size : _____   Form : _____

Date	Patient Name	Client ID	Initial Amount	Removed Amount	Remaining Amount	Authorized By	Dispensed By

Notes : _____

_____

_____

Bottle # : _____ Controlled Substance : _____

Serial # : _____ Class : _____

Expiration Date : _____ Concentration : _____

Container Size : _____ Form : _____

Date	Patient Name	Client ID	Initial Amount	Removed Amount	Remaining Amount	Authorized By	Dispensed By

Notes : _____

_____

_____

Bottle # : _____   Controlled Substance : _____

Serial # : _____   Class : _____

Expiration Date : _____   Concentration : _____

Container Size : _____   Form : _____

Date	Patient Name	Client ID	Initial Amount	Removed Amount	Remaining Amount	Authorized By	Dispensed By

Notes : _____

_____

_____

Bottle # : _____ **Controlled Substance :** _____

Serial # : _____ **Class :** _____

Expiration Date : _____ **Concentration :** _____

Container Size : _____ **Form :** _____

Date	Patient Name	Client ID	Initial Amount	Removed Amount	Remaining Amount	Authorized By	Dispensed By

Notes : _____

_____

_____

Bottle # : _____   Controlled Substance : _____

Serial # : _____   Class : _____

Expiration Date : _____   Concentration : _____

Container Size : _____   Form : _____

Date	Patient Name	Client ID	Initial Amount	Removed Amount	Remaining Amount	Authorized By	Dispensed By

Notes : _____

_____

_____

Bottle # : _____

Serial # : _____

Expiration Date : _____

Container Size : _____

Controlled Substance : _____

Class : _____

Concentration : _____

Form : _____

Date	Patient Name	Client ID	Initial Amount	Removed Amount	Remaining Amount	Authorized By	Dispensed By

Notes : _____

_____

_____

_____

Bottle # : _____ Controlled Substance : _____

Serial # : _____ Class : _____

Expiration Date : _____ Concentration : _____

Container Size : _____ Form : _____

Date	Patient Name	Client ID	Initial Amount	Removed Amount	Remaining Amount	Authorized By	Dispensed By

Notes : _____
_____
_____

Bottle # : _____ **Controlled Substance :** _____

Serial # : _____ **Class :** _____

Expiration Date : _____ **Concentration :** _____

Container Size : _____ **Form :** _____

Date	Patient Name	Client ID	Initial Amount	Removed Amount	Remaining Amount	Authorized By	Dispensed By

Notes : _____

_____

_____

Made in United States
North Haven, CT
06 February 2023

32125650R00070